SpringerBriefs in Publ

SpringerBriefs in Child Health

Series Editor
Angelo P. Giardino
Houston
Texas
USA

SpringerBriefs in Public Health present concise summaries of cutting-edge research and practical applications from across the entire field of public health, with contributions from medicine, bioethics, health economics, public policy, biostatistics, and sociology.

The focus of the series is to highlight current topics in public health of interest to a global audience, including health care policy; social determinants of health; health issues in developing countries; new research methods; chronic and infectious disease epidemics; and innovative health interventions.

Featuring compact volumes of 50 to 125 pages, the series covers a range of content from professional to academic. Possible volumes in the series may consist of timely reports of state-of-the art analytical techniques, reports from the field, snapshots of hot and/or emerging topics, elaborated theses, literature reviews, and in-depth case studies. Both solicited and unsolicited manuscripts are considered for publication in this series.

Briefs are published as part of Springer's eBook collection, with millions of users worldwide. In addition, Briefs are available for individual print and electronic purchase.

Briefs are characterized by fast, global electronic dissemination, standard publishing contracts, easy-to-use manuscript preparation and formatting guidelines, and expedited production schedules. We aim for publication 8-12 weeks after acceptance.

More information about this series at http://www.springer.com/series/10138

Julie A. Boom • Rachel M. Cunningham

Understanding and Managing Vaccine Concerns

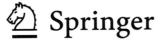 Springer

Julie A. Boom
Houston
Texas
USA

Rachel M. Cunningham
Houston
Texas
USA

ISSN 2192-3698   ISSN 2192-3701 (electronic)
ISBN 978-3-319-07562-4   ISBN 978-3-319-07563-1 (eBook)
DOI 10.1007/978-3-319-07563-1
Springer Cham Heidelberg New York Dordrecht London

Library of Congress Control Number: 2014940939

Printed on acid-free paper

Springer is part of Springer Science+Business Media (www.springer.com)

Contents

Chapter 1
Introduction

Abstract Despite the important role that vaccines have played in dramatically improving public health over the last century, parental concern regarding vaccine safety and effectiveness continues to increase. Subsequently, many parents are choosing to delay certain vaccines or refuse vaccination altogether, leaving their children at increased risk for vaccine-preventable diseases. Moreover, the communities in which these children live may also be affected due to the breakdown of herd immunity.

Keywords Vaccine concerns · Vaccine safety · Vaccine refusal

1.1 Introduction

Vaccines are one of the most important public health contributions of the 20th century and are responsible for the sharp decline in vaccine-preventable diseases (VPDs) in the United States. The incidence of most VPDs in the US has declined by 98-99 % (CDC 1999) (Table 1.1).

Despite strong scientific evidence demonstrating the safety and effectiveness of vaccines, parental concerns continue to increase (Smith et al. 2011; Flanagan-Klyss et al. 2005; Freed et al. 2010). As a result, more parents are choosing to delay or refuse vaccinations for their children (Smith 2011; Flanagan-Klyss 2005; Freed et al. 2010). Smith et al. (2011) found that 26 % of parents have delayed one or more vaccines and 8 % have refused one or more vaccines for their children. Parental vaccine concerns may include erroneous beliefs that vaccines contain harmful ingredients, overwhelm the immune system, or cause autism and other developmental disorders.

As a result of a parent's decision to delay or refuse vaccines, a child may become behind on their vaccinations and susceptible to VPDs. Evidence has clearly indicated that children whose parents choose to delay or refuse vaccines are at increased risk of VPDs (Feikin et al. 2006; Salmon et al. 2009). Vaccine delay or refusal also has implications for communities due to the effects on herd immunity. Herd immunity refers to the overall immunity of a given population and is based on two factors – the proportion of immune individuals in a given population and the subsequent protection these individuals provide susceptible persons. Individuals may be immune due to vaccination or immunity acquired after natural infection (Fine 2004). Vaccine delay or refusal increases the number of susceptible persons

J. A. Boom, R. M. Cunningham, *Understanding and Managing Vaccine Concerns*,
SpringerBriefs in Public Health, DOI 10.1007/978-3-319-07563-1_1,
© Springer International Publishing Switzerland 2014

Table 1.1 Vaccine-preventable diseases: post-vaccine percent decrease in morbidity

Disease	Pre-vaccine estimated annual morbidity[a]	2011 reported cases[b]	Percent decrease
Smallpox	29,005	0	100%
Diphtheria	21,053	0	100%
Measles	530,162	220	99.9%
Mumps	155,760	404	99.7%
Pertussis	185,120	18,719	89.9%
Polio (paralytic)	16,316	0	100%
Rubella	47,734	4	99.9%
Congenital rubella syndrome	151	0	100%
Tetanus	539	36	93.3%

[a] Ruosh SW, Murphy TV, Vaccine-Preventible Disease Table Working Group (2007) Historical Comparisons of morbidity and mortality for vaccine-preventable diseases in the United States. J Am Med Assoc 298(18):2155–2163
[b] CDC's Morbidity and Mortality Weekly Report (MMWR). 2012;60(53):1–20

and can lead to the breakdown of herd immunity. The medical community has found these trends extremely frustrating and worrisome as recent outbreaks have occurred in communities where disease has spread among unvaccinated individuals (CDC 2013; CDC 2011; CDC 2008).

The sharp decline in VPDs in the US can be largely attributed to changes in public health policies related to vaccine mandates for school entry. While all states permit medical and/or religious exemptions to school-required vaccines, more and more states have passed laws that allow for philosophical exemptions in response to the growing number of parents with vaccine concerns.

As a result of this increase in parental vaccine concerns and exemptions, providers need an in-depth understanding of why parents are hesitant or refuse to vaccinate their children. These situations require knowledge and skill as many vaccine-hesitant parents are highly educated themselves, and will ask their provider for further medical explanation or advice. This brief describes the history of vaccine concerns, current trends in vaccine hesitancy and refusal, and provides adaptable management strategies that providers can utilize in daily practice.

Chapter 2
History of Vaccine Concerns

Abstract Vaccine concerns date back to the eighteenth century during a time of smallpox epidemics in colonial America. Despite increased survival rates among those who were inoculated by variolation, opposition to this procedure was strong. Modern day vaccine fears were fueled by the Cutter Incident when incompletely inactivated polio vaccine was inadvertently administered to children resulting in significant morbidity and mortality. This incident was followed in the 1980s by the release of "*DPT: Vaccine Roulette*," a television documentary that engendered fears about the DTP vaccine and galvanized the formation of a well-known anti-vaccine group, National Vaccine Information Center. Parental vaccine safety concerns were fueled by this group and further strengthened with the publication of a controversial paper by Dr. Andrew Wakefield in which he suggested that the MMR vaccine was linked to autism. Despite the retraction of this paper and the discovery that many of its findings were fraudulent, others joined the anti-vaccine movement, including actress Jenny McCarthy and Dr. Bob Sears. These outspoken individuals have influenced many parents by suggesting that parents choose non-scientifically based alternative vaccination schedules that delay or omit vaccines.

Keywords Anti-vaccine · Dr. Bob · Jenny McCarthy · Barbara Loe Fisher · Andrew Wakefield · Edward Jenner · Cutter Incident · Vaccines

2.1 The Birth of the Anti-Vaccine Movement

Concerns surrounding vaccines date back to the eighteenth century during a time when colonial America experienced epidemics of smallpox. When smallpox entered a colonial port city as many as 60 % of residents became ill and an estimated 25 % died (National Humanities Center 2009). During one of these outbreaks in 1721, Dr. Zabdiel Boylston inoculated 280 people by rubbing material from a smallpox sore to a small wound (Bolyston 1726). This procedure was known as variolation. Boylston was met with strong resistance and soon there were two distinct groups—the "pro-inoculators" and the "anti-inoculators." The pro-inoculators group included Boylston and two clergy—Cotton Mather and Benjamin Colmon. The anti-inoculators were led by Dr. William Douglass, founder of the New England Currant, and James Franklin, the older brother of Benjamin Franklin. The

J. A. Boom, R. M. Cunningham, *Understanding and Managing Vaccine Concerns*,
SpringerBriefs in Public Health, DOI 10.1007/978-3-319-07563-1_2,
© Springer International Publishing Switzerland 2014

Table 2.1 Fatality of natural and inoculated smallpox (Boylston and Williams 2008)

	Boston[a]		England[b]	
	Died	Survived	Died	Survived
Natural smallpox	844	4915	2848	19,303
Inoculated smallpox	6	276	13	611[c]

[a] Relative risk natural vs. inoculated smallpox: 6.9 (range 3.2–15) $p<.0011$
[b] Relative risk natural vs. inoculated smallpox: 8.0 (range 4.7–13.6) $p<.0011$
[c] Relative risk inoculated in Boston vs. England: 1.02 (range 0.4–2.6) $p>0.9$

two groups publically shared heated exchanges in the Boston newspapers (National Humanities Center 2009).

In 1724, Boylston traveled to London where he published his findings on his work with smallpox inoculation (Boylston and Williams 2008). The findings were remarkable (Table 2.1). Boylston demonstrated that those in Boston who were not inoculated against smallpox had nearly 7 times the risk of dying from the disease and those in England who were not inoculated had 8 times the risk of death from smallpox (Boylston and Williams 2008).

Concerns about inoculations continued in England when Edward Jenner demonstrated that infecting a person with material from a cowpox blister could protect them from smallpox. His ideas were also met with strong opposition. At the time many people found the theory that intentional disease exposure could made a person healthier counterintuitive. Many believed it to be a violation of God's will because it changed the course of natural events. There were also fears that the vaccine itself would cause the disease and potentially death. Lastly, some opposed the idea of vaccination because of the belief that it violated their personal liberties. This opposition only increased as the British government implemented mandatory vaccination policies (Hammond et al. 2013).

In 1853, the British government passed a bill requiring all children to be vaccinated against smallpox by 6 months of age. Parents who failed to comply faced heavy fines or imprisonment. As a result, the first anti-vaccination movement was born. Richard, George, and John Gibbs founded the Anti-Compulsory Vaccination League in 1866 and the movement grew quickly with more than 200 anti-vaccination leagues formed in the following 30 years. The anti-vaccination movement in England was organized, strong, and sometimes violent. As a result of this movement, the British government passed a conscientious objection law in 1898. Soon after, immunization coverage rates drastically decreased as more than 200,000 certificates of conscientious objections were issued. Interestingly, however, Ireland and Scotland did not experience similar resistance, and subsequently saw a drastic reduction in smallpox, whereas England continued to experience high morbidity and mortality from the disease (Offit 2011).

2.2   The Cutter Incident

One concern about vaccines that has persisted throughout history is the perceived lack of safety. Unfortunately, the idea that vaccines could be unsafe was highlighted during the manufacturing of the polio vaccine. On the heels of one of the most significant public health achievements came one of the worst biological tragedies in the USA—the Cutter Incident. Cutter Laboratories was a small, family-owned pharmaceutical company in Berkeley, California that was licensed to produce Jonas Salk's polio vaccine. After years of scientific effort, Dr. Salk developed an inactivated polio vaccine. During the rush to mass produce the vaccine, Cutter laboratories released for administration several lots of vaccine in which the poliovirus was not fully inactivated but rather contained live, active poliovirus. 120,000 children were subsequently exposed to live, active poliovirus upon vaccination. Of those who received the vaccine, 70,000 suffered mild polio, 200 were permanently paralyzed, and 10 died. The company's error resulted in one of the worst pharmacologic disasters in US history and laid the groundwork for distrust in the pharmaceutical industry (Offit 2005, 2011).

2.3   The Twentieth Century Anti-Vaccine Movement

On April 19th, 1982, a NBC affiliate in Washington D.C. aired *"DPT: Vaccine Roulette,"* a one-hour documentary featuring the stories of children whose parents believed had been harmed by the DPT vaccine. DPT, also known as DTP, was a vaccine that protected against diphtheria, tetanus, and pertussis. Lea Thompson wrote, produced, and starred in the documentary which focused on the pertussis component of the vaccine. *"DPT: Vaccine Roulette"* featured vivid images of children with mental retardation, seizures, and other intellectual and physical disabilities. It also shared opinions from physicians who supported the belief that the DPT vaccine was unsafe and harmful. One physician, Dr. Robert Mendelsohn, stated "It's probably the poorest and most dangerous vaccine that we have now, [and] the dangers are far greater than any doctors have been willing to admit" (Offit 2011).

"DPT Vaccine Roulette" continued to make waves across the USA. It aired twice more in Washington D.C. as well as on NBC's *The Today Show*. Stories from the film were featured in magazines and newspapers across the country. One of the viewers was Barbara Loe Fisher. Fisher believed that her son had been irreparably harmed after receiving his fourth dose of DTP. Soon after the airing of *"DPT: Vaccine Roulette,"* Fisher and others formed "Dissatisfied Parents Together (DPT)." "Dissatisfied Parents Together" later became the well-known anti-vaccine group, the National Vaccine Information Center (NVIC), which remains a major source of vaccine misinformation in the USA. Fisher has been a fierce and unrelenting advocate and spokesperson for parents with vaccine concerns. Since the formation of

DPT and NVIC, she has voiced her concerns as the author of "*A Shot in the Dark: Why the P in the DTP Vaccination May Be Hazardous to Your Child's Health.*" Due to her influence in print and television media, she shaped many parents' beliefs about vaccines and raised nationwide interest in vaccine safety. In the years following the airing of "*DPT: Vaccine Roulette*" and the publication of "*A Shot in the Dark*," thousands of parents refused receipt of DPT. Moreover, vaccine manufacturers were suddenly flooded with personal injury lawsuits, which forced many companies to stop producing vaccines and led Congress to pass the National Childhood Vaccine Injury Act. This Act provided protection for vaccine manufacturers against litigation for vaccine injury and ensured the stability of the US national vaccination program (Offit 2011). An example of an early interview with Ms. Fisher on ABC's *The Morning Show with Regis Philbin* can be found at the following link (http://www.youtube.com/watch?v=-2b0-hMGm-o).

2.3.1 Andrew Wakefield

In 1998, Andrew Wakefield and colleagues at the Royal Free Hospital and School of Medicine in London published a case report of twelve children with ileal-lymphoid-nodular hyperplasia, non-specific colitis, and regressive developmental delay. This publication proposed that the MMR vaccine caused a series of events that included intestinal inflammation, loss of intestinal barrier function, entrance of encephalopathic proteins into the bloodstream, and subsequent development of autism. The intestinal biopsy findings in the twelve children supported his hypothesis (Wakefield et al. 1998). This paper was the nidus for a substantial increase in parental vaccine concerns, especially surrounding the MMR vaccine. Rates of MMR vaccine uptake decreased precipitously in England and measles outbreaks subsequently occurred throughout the United Kingdom.

Wakefield's paper triggered a flood of research that evaluated the theory that the MMR vaccine caused developmental delays, primarily autism. Following Wakefield's publication, numerous studies were conducted that compared groups of children who did and did not receive the MMR vaccine; no differences between the groups were identified (Taylor et al. 1999, 2002; Peltola et al. 1998; Dales et al. 2001; Farrington et al. 2001; Kaye et al. 2001; Madsen et al. 2002). In addition, in 2004, the Institute of Medicine reviewed the body of literature and found that the "evidence favors rejection of a causal relationship between the MMR vaccine and autism" (National Research Council 2014).

Wakefield's findings were later discovered to be fraudulent. In 2011, the investigative journalist Brian Deer summarized his inquiry into Wakefield's study in a series of articles published in the *British Medical Journal*. Through extensive interviews and research, Deer was able to uncover many concerning aspects of Wakefield's work. Deer's findings included the following: (1) the researchers failed to obtain institutional review board approval for the study; (2) study participants were recruited by an anti-vaccine group; (3) all of the children's medical histories were found to be misreported or altered; and (4) 8 months prior to the paper's publication Wakefield submitted a patent for a measles vaccine. Deer also discovered that Wakefield was retained by a personal injury lawyer representing several families who believed the MMR vaccine caused their child's autism and were suing pharmaceutical companies. The study was funded by the personal injury lawyer who referred his clients to Wakefield for participation with the intention of creating a case against the vaccine manufacturers. Soon after this information was released, ten of the thirteen authors withdrew their names from the paper (Offit 2011; Deer 2011).

In 2010, the *Lancet* formally retracted Wakefield's paper. Moreover, England's General Medical Council, the organization responsible for the licensure and registration of medical practitioners in the United Kingdom, found Andrew Wakefield guilty of multiple counts of dishonesty and stated that he had acted with "callous disregard" when he caused children to undergo clinically unnecessary invasive medical procedures. Wakefield was struck off the medical register in England and is no longer able to practice medicine there (Offit 2011; Deer 2011).

Soon after the MMR-autism association was debunked, anti-vaccine advocates turned their attention to vaccine ingredients, primarily thimerosal. Thimerosal is an ethylmercury preservative used in vaccines and other medications that is known to not cross the blood-brain barrier. Even though no scientific evidence has shown it to be harmful, as a precautionary measure in 1999, the US Public Health Service, American Academy of Pediatrics (AAP), and vaccine manufacturers agreed to remove thimerosal from most vaccines (AAP 1999). Today, the only vaccine containing thimerosal is the multi-dose influenza vaccine. However, anti-vaccine groups continue to perpetuate the belief that thimerosal in vaccines caused autism or was harmful. As a result, numerous peer-reviewed studies were conducted that examined whether receipt of a thimerosal-containing vaccine caused autism and no link was found (Stehr-Green et al. 2003; Madson et al. 2003; Fombonne et al. 2006; Hviid et al. 2003; Verstraeten et al. 2003; Heron and Golding 2004; Andrews et al. 2004). Also, in 2004, the Institute of Medicine reviewed the body of literature and found that the "evidence favors rejection of a causal relationship between thimerosal-containing vaccines and autism" (National Research Council 2014).

2.3.2   Jenny McCarthy

Over the last decade, anti-vaccine sentiment has become a cultural phenomenon. While Barbara Loe Fisher initiated the parent-led movement in the 1980s, it wasn't until 2007 that it became mainstream with the arrival of actress Jenny McCarthy as a celebrity spokesperson.

Soon after her son Evan was diagnosed with autism, McCarthy became convinced that vaccines were the cause. In 2007, during an appearance on *Oprah*, Jenny McCarthy shared the story of her son's descent into autism and publically blamed vaccines. McCarthy stated, "Right before my son got the MMR shot I said to the doctor, 'I have a very bad feeling about this shot. This is the autism shot, isn't it?' And he said, 'No! That is ridiculous. It is a mother's desperate attempt to blame something on autism.' And he swore at me. And then the nurse gave him that shot. And I remember going, 'Oh, God, no!' And soon thereafter I noticed a change. The soul was gone from his eyes" (Bratton 2011). Oprah followed with a response from the Centers for Disease Control and Prevention (CDC), which stated there was no science to support the connection between vaccines and autism. Jenny defiantly responded, "My science is Evan, and he's at home" (Bratton 2011).

McCarthy subsequently appeared on *Larry King Live, Good Morning America*, and several other television shows during which she repeatedly shared her son's story, criticized the public health and medical community, and lobbied against vaccines. Gradually McCarthy's message shifted from blaming the MMR vaccine to criticizing all vaccines, claiming that they contained toxins and that the recommended vaccination schedule called for too many vaccines too soon in a child's life. In 2008, McCarthy and then-partner, Jim Carrey, led a march and rally in Washington D.C. calling on medical and public health authorities to "green our vaccines" (Offit 2011). McCarthy's high-profile campaign against vaccines generated a significant amount of doubt and distrust among parents towards vaccines, the effects of which are still being felt today.

2.3.3 Dr. Bob Sears

At the same time that Jenny McCarthy was rallying against vaccines across the USA, a pediatrician from southern California wrote a best-selling book that gave credence to many myths about vaccines and offered vaccine-concerned parents alternative approaches to vaccination. Bob Sears, MD, is the son of Robert and Martha Sears, creators of the *Sears Parenting Library*, who for decades have dispensed advice on pregnancy, labor and delivery, breastfeeding, and parenting (Offit 2011). Dr. Bob, as he prefers to be called, has become the medical spokesperson for the anti-vaccine movement. Sears states that he is trying to find middle ground between parents with vaccine concerns and a medical community that continues to adamantly emphasize the safety of vaccines and the importance of timely vaccination. Sears' book, *"The Vaccine Book: Making the Right Decision for Your Child,"* is a collection of erroneous statements about vaccines, vaccine safety and efficacy, and vaccine-preventable diseases. Throughout his book, Sears minimizes the severity of vaccine-preventable diseases as well the susceptibility of under or unvaccinated children to these diseases. Moreover, he reinforces the practice of delaying or refusing vaccines so much so that he puts forth two vaccine schedules—Dr. Bob's alternative vaccination schedule and Dr. Bob's selective vaccination schedule. Both schedules modify the US recommended vaccination schedule; the alternative schedule delays specific vaccines until later ages whereas the selective schedule excludes the administration of some vaccines entirely (Sears 2011). The safety and effectiveness of these alternative vaccination schedules has not been studied by Sears or any other investigator. As Paul Offit, MD, so eloquently states, "It's…amazing when one considers that Robert Sears has never published a paper on vaccine science; never reviewed a vaccine license application; never participated in the creation, testing, or monitoring of a vaccine; and never developed an expertise in any field that intersects with vaccines—specifically, virology, immunology, epidemiology, toxicology, microbiology, molecular biology, or statistics. Yet he believes he can sit down at his desk and come up with a better schedule" (Offit 2011).

Chapter 3
Current Trends in Vaccine Hesitancy and Refusal

Abstract Increasing numbers of parents demonstrate high levels of vaccine concerns. Concurrently, increasing numbers of states allow personal belief exemptions for school required vaccinations. Unvaccinated individuals and communities with high rates of nonmedical vaccine exemptions are at greater risk for vaccine-preventable diseases. Rates of nonmedical vaccine exemptions have continually increased during the last two decades resulting in outbreaks of vaccine-preventable diseases such as measles and pertussis.

Keywords Exemptions · Vaccine refusal · Children · Vaccines · School health · Clustering · Outbreak potential · School mandate

3.1 Prevalence of Vaccine Hesitancy and Refusal

Despite overwhelming scientific evidence demonstrating the safety and effectiveness of vaccines, rates of vaccine hesitancy and refusal continue to increase, which potentially threatens the advances made in historically low rates of vaccine-preventable diseases (Smith 2011; Flanagan-Klyss 2005; Freed et al. 2010). While rates of VPDs remain at historic lows, recent outbreaks of pertussis and measles demonstrate the potential devastating effects of vaccine hesitancy and refusal.

A number of studies demonstrate that vaccine concerns and misconceptions are pervasive among parents, and occur even among those who immunize their children (Gellin et al. 2000; Gust et al. 2005; Freed et al. 2010). Freed et al. (2010) found that more than 50 % of parents reported having concerns about the adverse affects of vaccines, 25 % reported believing that some vaccines cause autism. Gellin et al. (2000) found that 23 % of parents agreed with the belief that children receive more immunizations than are good for them and 25 % were concerned that immunizations could weaken their child's immune system. A study by Shui et al. (2006) found that 21 % of parents reported being very concerned about vaccines.

Some parents demonstrate high levels of vaccine concern which can lead to the practice of delaying or refusing vaccines. Freed et al. (2010) reported that 11.5 % of parents previously refused at least one vaccine for their child, while Smith et al. (2011) found that approximately 39 % of parents delayed or refused a vaccine, 26 % delayed one or more recommended vaccines, and 8 % refused one or more vaccines.

J. A. Boom, R. M. Cunningham, *Understanding and Managing Vaccine Concerns*,
SpringerBriefs in Public Health, DOI 10.1007/978-3-319-07563-1_3,
© Springer International Publishing Switzerland 2014

In addition, 6% reported having both delayed and refused vaccines (Smith et al. 2011).

Pediatricians are experiencing the effects of these trends and increasingly report encountering parents with vaccine concerns. In a nationwide survey mailed to 1004 randomly selected AAP members, 85% reported having encountered parents who refused some vaccines in the previous year while 54% reported having encountered a parent who refused all vaccines (Flanagan-Klygis 2005). A study by Leib et al. (2011) of AAP members in Connecticut found that nearly 75% of pediatricians reported an increase in parental vaccine concerns and refusals in the last 10 years. Furthermore, more than 60% of participants reported having encountered at least one family in the previous year that refused all vaccines due to safety concerns (Leib et al. 2011).

3.2   Vaccine Exemptions

The increase in vaccine hesitancy and refusal is manifested by the rising rates of exemptions from school-required vaccines (Omer et al. 2006; Omer et al. 2009; Omer et al. 2012). Laws requiring vaccination date back to the introduction of the smallpox vaccine in the USA. The 1905 Supreme Court case *Jacobsen v. Massachusetts* affirmed the right of states to pass and enforce compulsory vaccination laws, and the 1922 Supreme Court case *Zucht vs. King* affirmed the constitutionality of school vaccine requirements (Omer et al. 2009). Laws requiring vaccination for school entry were an important part of a public health strategy to eliminate measles transmission among school-aged children in the latter half of the twentieth century. School-aged children carried the highest burden of disease for measles. Early evidence demonstrated that states with school vaccine mandates had dramatically lower rates of measles as compared to those without and, gradually, school requirements came to include additional vaccines such as hepatitis B, polio, and varicella (Orenstein and Hinman 1999). The success of the US vaccination program can largely be attributed to the implementation of such laws across all states (Orenstein and Hinman 1999; Omer et al. 2009).

All states permit medical exemptions from school-required vaccines. With the exception of Mississippi and West Virginia, all states permit religious exemptions as well (Orenstein and Hinman 1999; Blank et al. 2013). Increasing numbers of states are permitting personal belief exemptions, also known as philosophical or conscientious exemptions (Fig. 3.1). This type of exemption allows parents who are philosophically opposed to receipt of vaccination of one or more vaccines to opt out of school-required vaccines. Currently, 20 states have passed laws allowing personal belief exemptions (IAC 2013). In states without a personal belief exemption, religious exemptions are often used as a de facto philosophical exemption. Both religious and philosophical exemptions are considered nonmedical exemptions. One study by Salmon et al. (2005) found that 23% of nonmedical exemptions in Missouri, a state without a personal belief exemption, were self-reported by parents

Vaccine Exemptions

- – Philosophical
- – Religous
- – Medical

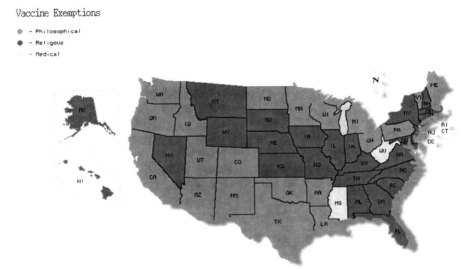

Fig. 3.1 Exemption type by state (Source: Johns Hopkins School of Public Health Institute for Vaccine Safety)

Fig. 3.2 Estimated percentages of children enrolled in kindergarten who have exempted from receiving one or more vaccines—USA, 2012–2013 school year. Exemptions might not reflect a child's vaccination status. Children with an exemption who did not receive any vaccines are indistinguishable from those who have an exemption but are up-to-date for one or more vaccines (CDC 2013)

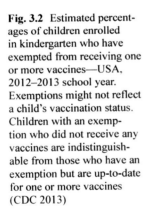

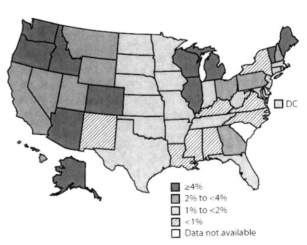

DC

- ≥4%
- 2% to <4%
- 1% to <2%
- <1%
- Data not available

to be due to religious reasons. These nonmedical exemptions serve as the primary measure for rates of vaccine refusal (Omer et al. 2009). As of 2013, approximately 2% of children in the USA were exempt from school-required vaccines. In some states rates exceed 5% (CDC 2013) (Fig. 3.2).

Exemption laws and procedures play an important role in maintaining low rates of VPDs. As personal belief exemptions have been introduced, utilization of such exemptions has increased. Between 1991 and 2004, the mean exemption rate for nonmedical exemptions in states that permit personal belief exemptions increased from 0.99 to 2.54%, averaging a 6% increase per year (Omer et al. 2006; Omer et al. 2009). States that allow personal belief exemptions have higher nonmedical exemption rates than those that only allow religious exemptions (Omer et al. 2006). Blank et al. (2013) found that the mean exemption rate for states that permitted personal belief exemptions was 2.8 versus 1.5 in states that only permit religious exemptions. Also, Omer et al. (2012) demonstrated that not only is the overall number of nonmedical exemptions increasing but also that they are increasing at an accelerated rate.

The process for obtaining a nonmedical exemption varies by state. Some states allow parents to exempt their child from vaccines by simply signing a prewritten statement on a school vaccination form whereas other states have a more difficult process and require parents to obtain a healthcare provider signature, undergo vaccine education, or notarize the exemption form. States with an easier exemption process tend to have higher exemption rates than those with a more difficult process (Omer et al. 2006; Blank et al. 2013). Of note, the state of Washington revised their exemption policies in 2011 to require parents requesting a nonmedical exemption to receive vaccine education by a licensed healthcare provider. Following the introduction of this policy change, the total exemption rate in Washington state decreased from 6.0% in the 2010–2011 school year to 4.5% in the 2011–2012 school year (Blank et al. 2013).

Evidence demonstrates that there are geographic areas in which families with similar attitudes and beliefs regarding vaccines cluster and the vaccine exemption rate is higher than average (Salmon et al. 1999; Smith et al. 2004; Birnbaum et al. 2013;). For example, the exemption rate in Oregon for the 2012–2013 school year was 6.4%, significantly higher than the national average of 1.8% (CDC 2013). A study by Ernst and Jacobs (2012) found large gaps in coverage across many states. For example, in Arizona, rates of personal belief exemptions varied by county from 0.7 to 8.5%. In Washington state, rates varied by county from 0 to 25.3% (Ernst and Jacobs 2012).

3.3 Implications of Vaccine Refusal

It is well-documented that children with nonmedical vaccine exemptions are at increased risk for contracting and transmitting vaccine-preventable diseases (Feikin et al. 2006; Salmon et al. 1999; CDC 2013; Atwell et al. 2013; Omer et al. 2008). Feikin et al. (2006) found that children in Colorado with nonmedical exemptions were 22 times more likely to contract measles and nearly six times more likely to contract pertussis than children who were immunized. Of note, 22% and 21% of children with measles and pertussis, respectively, acquired the infection in a school setting (Feikin et al. 2006). A study by Glanz et al. (2009) found that children whose parents refused vaccines were 23 times more likely to contract pertussis than vaccinated children. Between 1996 and 2007, 11% of pertussis cases were attributed

Fig. 3.3 US residents with measles who were unvaccinated ($n = 117$), by reasons for not receiving measles vaccine—USA, January 1– July 13, 2013. *: Includes persons who were unvaccinated because of their own or their parent's beliefs; †: Includes persons ineligible for measles vaccination, generally those aged < 12 months; §: Includes children aged 16 months—4 years who had not been vaccinated and international travelers ≥ 6 months who were unvaccinated but had no exemption; ¶: Includes persons who were known to be unvaccinated and the reasons were unknown (CDC 2013)

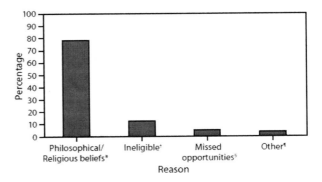

to parental vaccine refusal (Glanz et al. 2009). Similarly, intentionally unvaccinated children were 8.6 times more likely to contract varicella and 6.5 times more likely to contract pneumococcal disease/lobar pneumonia than their vaccinated peers (Glanz et al. 2010; Glanz et al. 2011). Salmon et al. (1999) found that children with nonmedical exemptions were 35 times more likely to contract measles than children who were vaccinated. Several measles outbreaks have occurred throughout the last few years. In 2013, a total of 159 cases of measles across 16 states were reported to the CDC. Of the 159 cases, 131 (82%) were in unvaccinated individuals, 92 (79%) of whom had personal belief exemptions to vaccines (CDC 2013) (Fig. 3.3). In 2011, 118 cases of measles were reported from January to May. Of these cases, 105 (89%) were in unvaccinated individuals, 24 of whom had claimed a nonmedical exemption (CDC 2011). Finally, in one of the most significant examples of the potential effects of vaccine refusal, the 2008 measles outbreak in San Diego was the result of an intentionally unvaccinated individual importing measles, subsequently infecting 11 others, and exposing more than 800 individuals (CDC 2008).

Beyond the individual risk of VPDs for exempt children, there is also a substantial community risk for outbreaks of VPDs in areas with high rates of nonmedical vaccine exemptions (Omer et al. 2008). The geographical clustering of children with vaccine exemptions has been associated with outbreaks of VPDs (Salmon et al. 1999; Atwell et al. 2013). In the 2008 San Diego measles outbreak, the intentionally unvaccinated individual attended a school with a nonmedical exemption rate of 9.6%, significantly higher than the national average (CDC 2008). A recent study by Atwell et al. (2013) demonstrated that the 2010 California pertussis outbreak was, in part, due to increased rates of nonmedical vaccine exemptions. Omer et al. (2008) found that census tracts in areas with high rates of nonmedical vaccine exemptions were three times more likely to also experience higher rates of pertussis incidence. In another study, Omer et al. (2006) found that states permitting personal belief exemptions had twice the rate of pertussis incidence as compared to those that only permitted religious exemptions. They also found that states with easier exemption processes were associated with a 90% increased pertussis incidence (Omer et al. 2006).

Chapter 4
Characteristics and Beliefs of Vaccine-Concerned Parents

Abstract Parents who delay or refuse vaccination tend to share common characteristics such as maternal age over 30, white race, higher income levels, and higher educational levels. These parents are also more likely to report distrust in their medical provider and more likely to seek care from a complementary and alternative medical (CAM) professional. Parents who delayed or refused vaccines are significantly less likely to believe vaccines are safe and effective. In addition, they are more likely to report misconceptions about vaccines such as beliefs about dangerous side effects, overload to the immune system, excessive number of doses, and causation of developmental disorders. In order to appropriately tailor vaccine education, it is important to understand the characteristics and beliefs of parents with strong vaccine concerns.

Keywords Vaccines · Vaccine refusal · Exemptions · Parents · Characteristics · Beliefs · Vaccine-hesitant · Vaccine-concerned

4.1 Characteristics of Vaccine-Concerned Parents

Several studies have identified similar risk factors for parents who are likely to delay or refuse vaccines. Smith et al. (2004) examined National Immunization Survey (NIS) data sets collected between 1995 and 2001 for children 19–35 months of age. Children who were unvaccinated were more likely to be white with a mother > 30 years of age who had a college degree. In addition, their family was more likely to have an income ≥ $75,000 and to have four or more children (Smith et al. 2004). Smith et al. (2011) re-examined NIS data in 2009 and found similar characteristics of children whose parents had delayed or refused a vaccine. Again, these children were more likely to be white with a married, English-speaking mother ≥ 30 years of age who had a college degree. Also, their family was more likely to have an income > 400 % of the federal poverty level, to be privately insured, and to have four or more children in their family (Smith et al. 2011). Additional studies have found similar findings (Gaudino and Robison 2012; Gust et al. 2008; Salmon et al. 2005). An analysis of parents in Colorado whose children contracted pertussis and who had previously refused pertussis vaccination revealed similar characteristics. These parents were more likely to be white, to be greater than 30 years of age, and of higher socioeconomic status based on median income (Glanz et al. 2009). Birnbaum et al.

J. A. Boom, R. M. Cunningham, *Understanding and Managing Vaccine Concerns*,
SpringerBriefs in Public Health, DOI 10.1007/978-3-319-07563-1_4,

(2013) and Richards et al. (2013) examined schools with high nonmedical exemptions rates in Arizona and California, respectively, and found that rates were highest in predominantly white schools.

Parents who delay or refuse vaccines are more likely to report having a poor relationship with their healthcare provider and have higher levels of distrust in the medical and public health community (Smith et al. 2011). They are also more likely to have higher levels of trust in CAM providers, higher rates of utilization of CAM providers, and more likely to report that their child's primary care provider is a CAM professional (Salmon et al. 2005).

4.2 Beliefs of Vaccine-Concerned Parents

Parents of both vaccinated and unvaccinated children commonly report concerns about vaccines, although parents who ultimately go on to refuse vaccines are more likely to express stronger concerns (Gaudino and Robison 2012). The ease with which parents can obtain a vaccine exemption may also be a contributing factor in the choice to refuse vaccines (Gaudino and Robison 2012, Omer et al. 2006).

Among concerned parents who chose to vaccinate despite strong concerns, the main reasons for doing so were the risk of disease, school and/or daycare requirements, and healthcare provider recommendation (Shui et al. 2006). Parents who delayed or refused vaccines are significantly less likely to believe vaccines are safe, effective, and necessary to protect their child's health (Smith 2011; Salmon et al. 2005). In addition, parents who delayed or refused vaccines are significantly more likely to report common misconceptions and concerns about vaccines, primarily that there are dangerous side effects, that they overwhelm the immune system, are given too closely together, and may cause autism and other developmental disorders (Smith 2011; Salmon et al. 2005). Among parents who declined vaccines, the reason most often cited for doing so was concerns about vaccine safety (Salmon et al. 2005). Additional risk factors identified among parents who exempt their child from school-required vaccines include knowing someone who believes vaccines injured their child, unconventional child birthing, and high distrust in healthcare providers (Gaudino and Robison 2012).

Chapter 5
Management Strategy for Vaccine-Concerned Parents: The C.A.S.E Approach

Abstract It is essential that the medical and public health communities respond to vaccine concerns and make every effort to maintain and improve vaccination coverage rates. As increasing numbers of providers encounter parents with vaccine concerns, they are faced with the challenge of how to best communicate with such parents while caring for their children. One method that has been suggested for organizing conversations with vaccine-concerned parents is the C.A.S.E approach.

Keywords Healthcare providers · Vaccines · Practice · C.A.S.E, · Patient management · Communication · Provider response

5.1 Communication Strategies

Providers remain the most influential and trusted source of information for parents with vaccine concerns (Gellin et al. 2000; Gust et al. 2005; Frederickson et al. 2004). It has been demonstrated that parents who previously expressed vaccine hesitancy or refused a vaccine became more amenable to vaccination following active listening and counseling from their healthcare provider (Frederickson et al. 2004; Gust et al. 2008). Parents who initially refused vaccines and later went on to vaccinate their child attribute their decision change to counseling and reassurance from their healthcare provider (Gust et al. 2008). While many parents may express concerns and questions about vaccines, they also believe that vaccines continue to be a good way to protect their children from disease and, ultimately, choose to vaccinate (Freed et al. 2010; Gust et al. 2005). Undoubtedly, providers play a critical role in parental vaccination decision-making.

5.2 The C.A.S.E Approach

One approach that has been suggested for organizing these conversations with parents is the C.A.S.E approach which was developed by Alison Singer, mother of a child with autism and President of the Autism Science Foundation (Jacobsen et al. 2013). The approach utilizes the acronym "C.A.S.E" which stands for the following: Corroborate, About Me, Science, Explain/Advise. After engaging the parent in an open dialogue and eliciting the specific concerns, Jacobsen et al. (2013) suggest that the provider begin by offering a corroborative statement. This statement would acknowledge the source of the parent's concerns without validating the concern itself. Next, the provider should introduce themselves as a subject matter expert and explain that they will provide evidence-based information. The provider should then transition into a discussion about the scientific evidence that addresses the parent's specific concerns. Finally, the conversation should culminate with the healthcare provider providing an evidence-based recommendation.

Utilizing the C.A.S.E approach in the clinical setting with vaccine-hesitant parents can provide structure for providers during what may seem like a daunting, and potentially out-of-control conversation. Great care should be given to choose words carefully as a verbal misstatement may take many more words to clarify or undo. In addition, these conversations cannot be rushed. If the family perceives that the provider is trying to hurry the conversation, it may be perceived as an attempt to cover something up or skirt an issue. For this reason, some providers may ask families with vaccine concerns to schedule a special appointment at the end of a day to allow for a longer, more in-depth conversation to occur.

Prior to applying the C.A.S.E approach, the provider must first carefully listen to the parent to elicit all of the vaccine concerns. When asked about vaccine concerns, the parent may respond with a single misconception or several concerns. At this point, however, it is important to make every attempt to elicit all of the parents' concerns. Otherwise, the provider will not have the opportunity to directly address all of the concerns, some of which may be brought up later in the conversation by the parent and used to bolster the parent's decision not to vaccinate. By eliciting all concerns in the beginning, the provider more clearly understands the parental perspective and potential controversy is limited. Also, if there is more than one caregiver in the room i.e. two parents or one parent and one grandparent, it is important to elicit concerns and discuss the issue with both caregivers. Often, one caregiver may influence the vaccine decisions even though that person may not be acting as the spokesperson in the exam room. The following is example of a strong introductory statement to elicit parental concerns:

Provider: *"You seem to have concerns about vaccinations. Will you share your thoughts with me?"* (Provider pauses to listen for initial response) *What other worries do you have with regard to the vaccine? I want to be sure that I understand all of your concerns."* (Provider gives parent the opportunity to express any additional thoughts) (Leask et al. 2012)

5.2.1   The C.A.S.E Approach—"Corroborate"

After listening to parental concerns, the provider should offer a corroborating statement to the parent. The purpose of the statement is to establish common ground between the provider and the parent. When offering this statement, it is important that it does not endorse the vaccine misinformation as truth. This is the most difficult step of the C.A.S.E approach as it can be difficult to find neutral statements. The following are examples of strong corroborative statements that can be used for a variety of vaccine issues:

"There certainly have been many stories about that in the news recently."

"You are not the first patient who has come to me with that concern."

"I have spoken with other parents who share your concerns in that area."

"The internet has a lot of information similar to that which you just shared with me."

"I saw that on TV too. That program raised concerns for some families."

"I read that article also. That article raised many of the concerns that you also have."

"Many of my patients have approached me with similar thoughts and questions."

"You have described a sincere concern for you and your family."

The following are examples of corroborative statements that may unintentionally endorse parental vaccine hesitancy:

"I saw that program on TV too. I can appreciate why you think that."

"After your experience, I would understand why you would want to avoid vaccination."

"I can see your point."

"Your concerns are real."

"I can certainly understand why you feel that way."

Corroborative statements generally don't need to be tailored for a specific vaccine concern. Therefore, a provider can adopt those that they are comfortable using in daily conversations with patients.

5.2.2   The C.A.S.E Approach—"About Me"

Often, families have already chosen a provider based on reputation in the community, advice from a friend, etc. Therefore, the parent seeks medical care from someone who they already respect and are ready to trust. When discussing vaccine concerns with parents, the provider needs to take the time to purposely build on the inherent trust and respect that serve as the foundation for the patient-provider relationship. Providers should offer one or two simple statements that will convey to the parent the level of their magnitude of medical knowledge in the area of vaccines. When offering these statements, providers need to remember that they are one of the most important influences on parental vaccine decision-making (Gellin et al. 2000; Gust et al. 2005; Frederickson et al. 2004). A study by Gust et al. (2003) found that 89 % of parents agreed with the statement "I usually follow my child's doctor's advice." Examples of personal statements that a provider could make include:

"I studied this issue extensively during my medical training and have continued to stay abreast of these issues."

"I have dedicated many hours of my personal time studying this issue."

"I recently attended a CME conference where this topic was addressed at length."
"This is an area of interest of mine, therefore, I read the medical literature in this area extensively."
"I recently attended a medical meeting where expert speakers addressed many of the questions that you have."

Of course, a provider should reflect on their own interests and knowledge base and craft statements that would best describe their background in this area. Although it may seem like bragging, it is not. The family will not appreciate your dedication to knowledge in this area unless you make it a point to share it with them.

Occasionally, the "about me" statement offers the provider other opportunities to find common ground between the parent and the provider. For instance, the parent may have expressed their struggle to make what they feel are stressful decisions on behalf of their child. In this case, the provider might decide to share that in addition to their medical expertise that he/she is also a parent or grandparent. The provider can further explain how they have vaccinated their own children. The provider will need to use their judgment to determine if the personal information might benefit or potentially harm the discussion. Some providers may not feel comfortable sharing their personal situations with their patients. In that case, this can easily be skipped. Parents will rarely ask about a provider's personal situation, but occasionally will feel more engaged and place more trust in a provider who has shown a willingness to share a brief piece of their personal life. For some parents, actions will speak louder than words and they want to hear that their doctor practices what they preach.

5.2.3   The C.A.S.E Approach—"Science"

Following the "about me" statement, the provider will then directly address each of the vaccine concerns raised by the parents. Providers must be well versed in the medical literature to complete this step efficiently and confidently. The tone and delivery of the message is also important. Parents will pick up on subtle cues and may interpret minor hesitations as indecision on behalf of the provider. If one concern has been voiced as most important, address that concern first. These statements need to be specifically tailored to address the exact concern raised. The following are common vaccine concerns raised by parents and example statements that could be used by providers to address them (Tables 5.1 and 5.2).

Any of the statements in the table might be asked to a provider with varying degrees of sophistication. Providers need to be able to answer these questions using simple nonmedical language at various educational levels which can be difficult and require some prior thought. However, given the advanced educational background of many vaccine-hesitant parents, providers also need to be able to explain these issues at a college or graduate level (Smith et al. 2011; Smith et al. 2004; Salmon et al. 2005; Richards et al. 2013; Atwell et al. 2013). To do this, they need to remain abreast of the most recent literature with regard to general vaccine concerns and specific vaccine issues. Up-to-date vaccine information can be found at the following websites: www.cdc.gov/vaccines, www.immunize.org, www.immunizationinfo.org.

Table 5.1 Examples of provider responses to common general vaccine concerns

Parental concern:	Provider response:
"I'm worried vaccines will make my baby autistic. My nephew has autism."	*"There are numerous large medical studies examining a scientific link between vaccines and autism. No link has been found. In addition, the United States Institute of Medicine examined all of these studies and has also found no link between any vaccine and autism. We know that in some cases, autism is due to a genetic cause. In many other cases, we don't yet understand the cause. Medical providers and scientists around the world are working to understand the cause and cure for autism. We don't want one more child to be diagnosed with autism. That said, vaccines have been thoroughly studied and they are not the cause. You can vaccinate your baby today confident that the vaccines will not cause autism."* (Offit and Moser 2011)
"I'm worried that babies are being given too many shots too early in life. They are simply too young."	*"I understand you want to protect your baby but it's important for you to understand that we give babies vaccines when they need them the most. The vaccines that we give babies are the ones that will prevent them from dying when they are infants. They have been tested in infants and been found safe and effective at these very young ages of 2, 4, and 6 months. So you don't need to worry that it's too many too soon. In fact, I would worry if we didn't give all of these vaccines to your baby on time because these diseases are worrisome—Hib, pneumococcal, pertussis."* (Offit and Moser 2011)
"So many vaccines will weaken my child's immune system."	*"Your baby's immune system is ready to respond from the moment they are born. The vaccines we give your baby are just a very small fraction of the 'work' that their immune system will do during their childhood. Every time your baby gets a virus or simple illness like a cold your baby's immune system does much more 'work' than it does after multiple vaccinations. Because we use much more scientifically refined vaccines today than we were able to use 20 to 30 years ago, your baby's vaccines require much less effort from their immune system than even the vaccines that you received."* (Offit and Moser 2011)
"My oldest child got all of his shots on time and now he has asthma. I think that all of the shots early in life may have caused it as it doesn't run in our family."	*"You did the right thing by vaccinating your child on time—it was absolutely the right thing to do. I know your child's asthma is a struggle for you now. That said, the vaccines and your child's asthma are unrelated. We often look for an explanation for things that happen to us in our lives and sometimes we try to make connections between one event and another. This is an example of two things that happened to*

Table 5.1 (continued)

Parental concern:	Provider response:
	your child that were completely medically unrelated. Scientists have looked at this and proven that there is no link between vaccines and any chronic illness like asthma. It's important that you continue to vaccinate your child knowing that the vaccines are not harmful and in fact, are very important in protecting your son's health. He needs to receive a flu vaccine every year as children with asthma can get very sick from the flu." (Offit and Moser 2011)
"My husband and I are planning to exempt our child from vaccines at the time of shcool entry."	*"I know you and your husband want to do everything you can to protect your child from any type of harm. But not vaccinating them is actually opening up the door to harm. First, you can't rely on the vaccines that other children have received because vaccines don't work perfectly all of the time. The child sitting beside them at school may have been vaccinated but if they are in the small percentage of children in which the vaccine didn't work they could inadvertently transmit a disease to your child. Also, nowadays, there are lots of kids at school that may not have been able to be vaccinated. Some children with immune problems or who have had other bad illnesses may not be able to receive vaccines. They too could transmit a disease to your child. It's important to understand that if your child gets sick that your child could make a vulnerable child sick also. Unfortunately, vaccination decisions are decisions that we make as parents that not only affect our child but also affect the other children around them. Vaccines are what allow our children to gather in schools, places of worship, parties, and not worry that they will make each other sick. So even though your thinking may make sense at first thought it violates the social contract that we all hold with each other"* (Offit and Moser 2011).
"I have read about thimerosal and I don't want my child to receive any vaccines that have thimerosal in them."	*"That is not a problem at all. Even though there is no data to show thimerosal is harmful it was taken out of almost all vaccines in the early 2000s. All of the infant and kindergarten doses are available without thimerosal. There are multiple flu shots without thimerosal also. "If at any point we need to give your child a shot that has thimerosal in it...". Thimerosal is a type of mercury that is very different than the type that you were told to avoid during your pregnancy, methylmercury. This type will not harm your developing child's brain"* (Offit and Moser 2011; ACOG 2014)

Table 5.2 Examples of provider responses to specific vaccine concerns

Parental concern:	Provider response:
DTaP: *"I don't want my baby to receive the pertussis portion of the vaccine. It is harmful and doesn't work that well"*	*"The pertussis vaccine is one of the most important vaccines that your baby will receive. Pertussis, or whooping cough, is a very dangerous disease, especially in children less than 1 year. About 4 out of 5 deaths occur in babies less than 3 months of age. Babies can have high rates of pneumonia from pertusssis. All of the coughing prevents the baby from being able to breathe in—so the baby doesn't get enough oxygen. These babies can turn blue; some also have seizures and other brain problems as a result of the infection. We know that the current vaccine that we use, DTaP, doesn't make as long lasting immunity as we need. So, your child will need booster doses as they get older. The vaccine will give your baby the best protection that we have to offer, though, as an infant. So we really need to vaccinate today. We don't want to risk letting your baby get this disease."* (CDC 2012)
IPV: *"No one in the United States gets polio anymore so I don't want to give that vaccine to my baby."*	*"You are right. We don't see polio in the United States anymore, but that is because of the vaccine! We continue to vaccinate children because polio is still in several countries including Afghanistan, Pakistan and Nigeria. This virus is spread person-to-person, so it is just a plane ride away. I wouldn't want you to take any chance that your baby could possibly become crippled from this horrible germ."* (CDC 2012)
Hib: *"My husband and I are delaying all vaccines until 2 years of age. As this one isn't required by our state for kindergarten, we have decided to avoid it all together. We want to minimize putting any unnecessary substances into my baby as much as possible."*	*"I certainly support your interest in minimizing putting unnecessary substances into your baby's body. For that reason, I will always give you my best recommendations for promoting good nutrition, trying to keep your baby's environment safe and only using antibiotics when they are necessary. I want to assure you that vaccines are one of the very necessary things that your baby's body needs to remain healthy. The Hib bacteria especially affects infants and toddlers and can cause infection of the covering of the brain called meningitis. Before we had a vaccine against this germ, many children had hearing loss from this; some children died. I wouldn't want you to take any chances that your baby could suffer from this. It isn't required for kindergarten entry in some states because most children older than 5 years are likely naturally immune. I want to stress again- vaccination against Hib for babies is necessary and is the healthy choice for your baby"* (CDC 2012).
Hepatitis B: *"It seems unnecessary to me to give this vaccine to my baby. I know that my tests for this were negative. We will raise our baby in a way that he will not adopt risky behaviors."*	*"Hepatitis B vaccine is very important for all infants to receive. I hear that you are negative. But because these blood tests can sometimes be confusing to understand, the mother's blood tests can be misinterpreted. Just by giving the vaccine alone, we can prevent this infection from traveling from mother to baby 70–95% of the time. So, this vaccine acts as an important safety net for everyone. As your child's doctor, I want to be part of the team that will help counsel your child his whole life against risky behaviors. That said, I know that this vaccine could help prevent liver cancer someday if you and I aren't around at the time that he does choose to adopt a risky behavior."* (CDC 2012)

Table 5.2 (continued)

Parental concern:	Provider response:
Rotavirus: *"It seems to me that a 2 month old is too young to receive a live vaccine. It just seems risky."*	*"When we say that a vaccine is "live," that can sound scary but it isn't. This is what it means. The virus isn't fully killed but has been weakened so much that it can't make you sick. It still works inside your body to make an immune response. This vaccine was tested in a large population of infants—it is very safe and works very well too. It protects your baby against a very bad virus that causes lots of diarrhea and vomiting. Even though your baby is unlikely to die from this in the US, many babies to go to the ER because they get behind on fluids from all of the diarrhea and vomiting. Almost all children get this by age 5 years if they aren't vaccinated—so you really can't escape this virus. Believe me—this is a virus you want to avoid– the vaccine is the best choice."* (CDC 2012)
Rotavirus: *"I've read on the internet that this vaccine might cause intussusception. I think that just getting the virus and having the diarrhea would be much safer overall."*	*"Actually, experts have looked into just what you are taking about. The older vaccine was taken off the market in the late 1990s for just this reason. The newest information has shown that this can still occur but is much more rare with the vaccines that we use today. Even with this slight increased risk of intussusception (telescoping of the intestines), the risk to your child from rotavirus if he goes unvaccinated is much higher than the risk of intussusception after vaccination. We can stay in close contact after your baby receives the vaccine if you like just in case you have any concerns"* (Glass and Parashar 2014)
MMR: *"I've heard that this vaccine causes autism. My friends have all delayed giving it to their children until 2 years or later. That is my plan."*	*"Unfortunately, there a doctor in the U.K. that tried to spread this myth, but it's not true at all. Since then, tons of research has shown that there is no link between any vaccine and autism. Unfortunately, that doctor's misstatements made a lot of parents worry. You can rest assured that the MMR vaccine won't cause your baby harm. In fact, it is more important now, more than ever, that your child receives it on time. Because so many parents in the U.K. that haven't vaccinated, we have children and adults traveling bringing measles disease to us. So to protect your baby, we need to vaccinate today"* (Offit and Moser 2011).
Varicella: *"I think that it would be better for my child to get the natural disease. My siblings and I all got the chickenpox at the same time and we are all fine. In fact, my daughter's playgroup is thinking about holding a chickenpox party if one of the kids comes down with it."*	*"Even though you and I had chickenpox when we were young, it wasn't without risk. Chickenpox is risky because it opens up your skin to bacterial infection in hundreds of places all over your body. It can also infect your lungs. Before we had the vaccine, about 70 kids and adults died from the illness every year. One of the benefits of growing up now compared to when we grew up is having the availability to have vaccines such as this one. The vaccine also decreases your child's chance of getting shingles later in life which is when chickenpox reactivates when you're older. I understand your playgroup has discussed this and that the thoughts of your peers are important to you and I respect that. That said, chickenpox parties put everyone's children at risk for this dangerous disease. Instead, we need to make sure everyone in the playgroup is vaccinated"* (CDC 2012; Offit and Moser 2011).

Table 5.2 (continued)

Parental concern:	Provider response:
Hepatitis A: *"We rarely eat at restaurant and have no plans of traveling with our baby out of the country. I don't understand why our baby would need this vaccine."*	*"Even though hepatitis A is rarely deadly, the virus makes children and adults very ill. Children are at risk for getting the virus from an infected adult in the home. Children can be exposed in childcare settings. Children sometimes don't show symptoms or aren't diagnosed and then spread the infection to adults. By vaccinating children, we protect adults and prevent outbreaks in our communities"* (CDC 2012).
Influenza: *"The last time I got a flu shot, I got sick. I'm not going to risk that with my child."*	*"When you receive the flu vaccine, your body is exposed to a very small piece of the dead virus that cannot make you sick. Your immune system responds to this microscopic piece of virus and generates an immune response. So, the next time your body is exposed to the virus, it will fight the virus off and it won't make you sick. About a third of people report that they don't feel well with either muscle aches, fever or fatigue after getting just a simple injection with sterile water. So, we know that feeling under the weather after any injection can happen—but it is not caused by the vaccine. Sometimes too, you may have been exposed to a virus like the common cold virus in the day or two just before your vaccine. You then get vaccinated and it makes you think that the vaccine caused the illness. In actuality, another virus, not the vaccine, caused the illness."*
Influenza: *"My child got the flu shot last year just as you suggested and got the flu months later. I just don't think that the vaccine works."*	*"It is important to remember that the flu isn't just the common cold. The flu can cause severe illness that can result in hospitalization. Over each of the past few years, approximately 160 pediatric deaths have occurred in the United States. The shot form of the vaccine prevents approximately 7 out of 10 children from getting moderately or severely ill. The nasal spray prevents over 8 of 10 children from moderate or severe disease. You want to take every opportunity that you can to decrease your chance of getting this bad virus. The current flu vaccines offer the best possible protection against this potentially severe illness"* (CDC FluView)
Influenza: *"I am fine giving the flu shot, but not the flu vaccine in the nose. I've heard that the one is the nose is alive and that sounds too strong for my child."*	*"The nasal flu vaccine isn't too strong at all. The virus in the vaccine has been changed so it can't reproduce itself at regular body temperatures. The vaccine works very well, especially in children. Kids can avoid a needle in their arm too. The vaccine can cause a stuffy nose, but most of my patients don't complain too much about that."*
HPV: *"We have talked about the HPV vaccine and our daughter doesn't need it. We are teaching abstinence until marriage."*	*"Unfortunately, the risk of HPV isn't that simple. By the age of 50, 4 out of 5 US women have been exposed to the HPV virus. The virus can even be contracted just by skin-to-skin contact. We don't understand why some people clear this infection and why it goes on to cause cancer in others, but it does. It is possible that your child could remain abstinent until marriage, but their future spouse might have had one prior partner. Just through one prior exposure, the spouse may bring this to the marriage. Years into the marriage, your daughter could have a bad Pap smear and be diagnosed with cancer. We can avoid all of this worry by giving the vaccine"* (CDC 2012)

Table 5.2 (continued)

Parental concern:	Provider response:
HPV: *"I'm worried that if we give our daughter the HPV vaccine that she will become more interested in sex or start having sex."*	*"The vaccine will not make her sexually active. He/she will receive the shot at the same visit that we give the teenage Tdap and meningitis vaccines. Your child won't be able to distinguish the HPV vaccine from the other vaccines that we give at this age. Giving a child a shot doesn't change their behavior. We give the tetanus shots and children don't start trying to step on rusty nails! The same goes for this vaccine; your child will be no more or less interested in sexual activity because of the shot. Just in case you're interested, some scientists have even proved this."* (Mayhew et al. 2014)
Meningitis: *"I've heard about this disease in the news and some recent cases in college students. This disease is so rare and the current vaccine doesn't even protect against all of the types that college kids get—isn't the media blowing it out of proportion?"*	*"Meningitis is a disease that you don't want to take any chances with. Even though it is rare, the disease is devastating. Teens get sick very fast and can end up critically ill and can die. When it does strike, it happens so fast that there's almost nothing that can be done. This is one case where the media isn't blowing it out of proportion—this is a scary disease that we can prevent. I don't want you to wait to vaccinate until there is a case of meningitis at your child's school. The time to vaccinate it now"* (Offit and Moser 2011).

5.2.4   The C.A.S.E Model—"Explain/Advise"

At this final step of the conversation, the provider needs to offer an action to the parent that he/she would like the parent to adopt. The provider should be bold and not hesitate to ask that the parent to take the action that the provider knows is medically sound. If the family senses hesitation at this stage, the parent may back away from taking the action that they were contemplating. The provider should include a time request in the action statement to avoid ambiguity. Strong explain/advise statements use presumptive formats which state a clear position on vaccination. These statements purposely limit participation and are more difficult to resist (Opel et al. 2013). The following are examples of strong explain/advise statements:

"Now that we've had a chance to discuss your concerns, let's vaccinate your baby today."

"It's important to not let another day go by without these important vaccines. We should give vaccines today and have you come back in 4 week intervals until your baby is completely caught up."

"As the vaccines need several weeks to begin to give your child immunity, let's get that process started as soon as possible to give your baby the most benefit. Let's vaccinate today."

"As this vaccine is the first in a three part series, let's go ahead and give the first dose today so your child can see the benefit of this vaccine that much sooner."

"We don't want any more time to elapse that your baby goes unprotected. Let's give all of the recommended vaccines today."

Weaker statements would include:
"Given our discussion, would you like to vaccinate today?"
"What do you think now that we have discussed your concerns?"
"After our discussion, are you still thinking that you don't want the vaccines?"

These weaker statements utilize participatory language in which the parent is questioned regarding interests, intentions, or beliefs about vaccines. In a cross-sectional observational study that included many vaccine-hesitant parents, parents were more likely to resist vaccine recommendations if the provider initiated the vaccine discussion using participatory language rather than presumptive language. In addition, almost half of the parents who initially resisted the providers recommendation shifted to accept it if the provider continued to pursue their original recommendation (Opel et al. 2013). Therefore, it is important to use strong presumptive statements that reinforce the original recommendation.

The provider should listen carefully to the parent's responses. Some parents will opt to follow the provider's advice and vaccinate. At that point, nursing staff should be informed of the parent's concern so they can reinforce any important information that may arise during or after the vaccine administration process. The provider should remain readily available in case additional questions arise. Some parents may move away from their original concern, but will instead begin to offer contingency statements that would still allow them to hedge and avoid vaccination at the current visit (Opel et al. 2014). Commonly used contingency statements include:
"I need to talk to the baby's father and he is not available right now."
"I don't think that I'm ready for it today but I'll come back next week."
"We're going away next week and I don't want there to be any possibility that the vaccines will ruin our trip."

Despite all of these efforts, some parents will continue to refuse while remaining committed to their original concern or belief about the vaccine. In these instances, the provider has not failed. These parents may have come to the appointment not remotely considering vaccination. In these cases, it is unrealistic to expect that the parent will move from refusal to active vaccine acceptance in one visit (Leask et al. 2012). Providers need to guard against the stress and emotional burden that caring for these patients may cause (Kempe et al. 2011).

Anecdotally, we have found the C.A.S.E approach to be a helpful, easily customizable tool to guide conversations with vaccine-hesitant parents. While many of these conversations may result in a shift in parental vaccine beliefs or behaviors, some will not. Some parents will remain steadfast in their choice not to vaccinate. In these instances, other management strategies should be considered.

Chapter 6
Additional Management Options

Abstract Despite sincere, informative conversations with vaccine-hesitant parents, some parents will choose to stand firm and delay or refuse vaccination. Undoubtedly, managing parents who delay or refuse vaccines is difficult. Providers need to understand the ethical issues involved as they implement alternative management strategies with these families.

Keywords Healthcare providers · Vaccines · Treatment refusal · Dismissal · Ethics · Communication

6.1 Ethical Considerations

The key ethical principles surrounding vaccine refusal discussions are autonomy, a person's right to determine the course of action most appropriate for him, and beneficence, the responsibility to help others. In the USA, parents are legally regarded as the best persons to determine the best course of action for their children (Goldstein 1977). In addition to parental autonomy, family privacy is also honored. Although these parental rights offer parents broad decision-making authority over their children, these rights become limited if their child's well-being is at risk (Opel et al. 2014). Providers also have a duty to protect vulnerable children from harm or neglect. To apply these principles to vaccine refusal, all possible risks and benefits of all of the various vaccine options must be considered to determine if vaccine refusal poses enough risk to result in serious harm to the child (Diekema 2004). During times of routine disease prevalence, it is unlikely that the risk of harm to the child would be serious enough to justify overriding parental autonomy (Opel et al. 2014; Diekema 2005). This risk analysis could shift, however, during an outbreak depending on the prevalence of disease and associated potential for harm. Under the principle of beneficence, providers have the responsibility to help others. Parents and providers may find common ground by discussing that they both are working to ensure that the child's welfare is maintained (Fernbach 2011). While providers must respect parental autonomy, provider autonomy should also be appreciated. Kamin

J. A. Boom, R. M. Cunningham, *Understanding and Managing Vaccine Concerns,* 31
SpringerBriefs in Public Health, DOI 10.1007/978-3-319-07563-1_6,
© Springer International Publishing Switzerland 2014

(2012) stated that, "Physicians should not be forced to provide care they think is wrong." The complex balance of these ethical issues may raise tensions between patients and providers.

6.2 Additional Communication Strategies

When discussing vaccine choices with parents, providers can employ several communication strategies. In order to effectively communicate, providers may need to use additional techniques to shift parental vaccine beliefs. Providers may need to explain the risks of not vaccinating in a way that is more understandable and real to the family. Providers and parents are likely to understand risks differently. During medical training, providers are typically taught about health risk in quantitative terms such as percentages, probability and prevalence. Data has shown, however, that most lay persons do not correctly interpret this data when it is presented to them (Schwartz et al. 1997). David Ropeik (2006) said it best in his Time magazine article, "You would think we'd get pretty good at distinguishing the risks likeliest to do us in from the ones that are statistical long shots. But you would be wrong. We agonize over avian flu, which to date has killed precisely no one in the USA, but have to be cajoled into getting vaccinated for the common flu, which contributes to the deaths of 36,000 Americans each year." Although presenting clinical evidence in terms of mathematical risk may seem more logical and persuasive to the provider, it may fail to present a complete picture to the patient. Sharing a personal story of a child who was affected by a vaccine-preventable disease or sharing written materials that relays personal stories may result in a more favorable outcome. These alternative methods help connect theoretical risk into more relatable possibilities (Cunningham and Boom 2013). One example of vaccine-related storytelling can be found in "*Vaccine-Preventable Disease: The Forgotten Story.*" This booklet contains 20 stories of individuals and families affected by a vaccine-preventable disease (Fig. 6.1).

In addition to storytelling, providers can explain how other families who are similar to them vaccinate their children. Given the prevalence of vaccine-hesitancy messages in the community, some parents may fail to realize that most parents choose to fully vaccinate their children (CDC 2013). Providers may choose to disclose how they vaccinate their own children. Finally, if parents are refusing all vaccines, persuading the parent to accept one vaccine might help build personal knowledge of positive experiences with vaccines and build trust in them. Some providers may not consider this a viable alternative arguing that permitting any degree of vaccine refusal conveys to the parent that vaccines aren't really that important (Opel et al. 2014). Others may argue that ultimately administering some vaccines are better than none (Offit and Moser 2009).

Fig. 6.1 Story of Haleigh
Throgmorton from "*Vaccine-
Preventable Disease: The
Forgotten Story*"

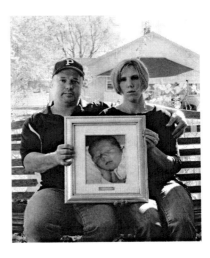

When Haleigh Throgmorton was a few weeks old, Rodney caught what resembled a cold.
Shortly after, Haleigh began coughing also—so severely that she was hospitalized. Doctors diagnosed both Rodney and Haleigh with pertussis ("whooping cough"), a vaccine-
preventable disease that is mild for adults but particularly dangerous for infants and young
children. At only 6 weeks old, Haleigh died. "Haleigh was too young to receive the vaccine," Rodney says. "It would have saved her life."

6.3 Dismissal

Following a conversation about vaccines, some providers may feel bewildered,
frustrated, and sometimes even angry that the parent is not choosing the medically
sound option for their child. Providers may feel that the patient/physician relationship has been undermined and trust is no longer present in the relationship. As a
result, the provider may choose to dismiss the family from their practice. Flanagan-
Klygis et al. (2005) define patient dismissal, or "firing", as "a last resort when all
other attempts at patient compliance have failed or difficult patient behavior makes
it impossible to maintain a relationship." A provider is within their rights to dismiss
a family so long as it is done properly. The provider must notify the family with
ample time to select another provider for their child (Diekema 2005). The AAP sug-
gests that these instances should be rare and pursued only after a concerted effort to
collaborate with the family (Diekema 2005).

Increasing numbers of providers are choosing to dismiss families who refuse
vaccines. In one study, 30 % of physicians reported asking families to leave their
practices based on refusal to vaccinate their children (Leib et al. 2011). Moreover,
more than 40 % of the providers who participated in this study agreed with the policy to dismiss families who refuse all vaccines (Leib et al. 2011). Flanagan-Klygis
et al. (2005) found that 28 % of AAP members would dismiss parents who refused

some vaccines and 39% would dismiss parents who refused all vaccines. Reasons given for dismissal include lack of trust, fear of litigation, and lack of shared goals. Vaccines are considered standard medical care and many of the pediatricians surveyed considered vaccine refusal as sub-standard medical care (Lieb et al. 2011). Many providers who opt to dismiss families from their practice perceive refusal to vaccinate as a form of neglect. In addition, some providers will choose not to care for unvaccinated children as they might pose a risk to other children in the practice (Gilmour et al. 2011; CDC 2008).

Some practices have also posted signs in their office that clearly state their policies regarding vaccination to ensure that parents who refuse vaccines are adequately informed from their very first visit.

6.4 Continuance of Care

Conversely, other providers will continue to care for these families arguing that unvaccinated children are in the most need of quality medical care (Lieb et al. 2011). The American Academy of Pediatrics (AAP), the American Medical Association (AMA) and the Centers for Disease Control and Prevention (CDC) discourage providers from dismissing families who may be choosing to delay or refuse vaccines (Diekema 2005; American Medical Association 2007; CDC 2012). The AAP encourages listening carefully to parental concerns while recognizing that parents and providers may weigh risk/benefit evidence very differently. They suggest that maintaining the relationship is essential to allow for additional vaccine discussions to occur at future visits with the hope that parents might reconsider vaccination at a later date (Diekema 2005; Diekema 2012). Dismissing families who refuse vaccines prevents additional opportunities for vaccine counseling from occurring. It also creates a risk for the child for disrupted care or for their parents to turn to an alternative medical provider who may be more likely to promote vaccine concerns (Diekema 2013).

Providers should remember that they are the most important resource for parents regarding vaccine decisions (Gellin et al. 2000; Gust et al. 2005; Frederickson et al. 2004). In one study, parents who accepted vaccines after initial vaccine refusal reported doing so based on conversations with their provider (Gust et al. 2008). Continuing to care for children whose parents refuse vaccines creates future opportunities to build trust and perhaps produce a more favorable outcome.

6.5 Liability Concerns

Providers may state that they fear liability risks should an unvaccinated child contract a vaccine-preventable disease. These risks can be minimized by carefully documenting the benefits of vaccination and risks of delaying or refusing vaccination. In addition to standard documentation, the provider may ask the parent to sign a refusal to vaccinate waiver. The AAP has provided sample waivers which can be found at http://www2.aap.org/immunization/pediatricians/pdf/refusaltovaccinate. pdf. This additional step may help ensure that parents understand the consequence of their vaccine decisions (Schwartz and Caplan 2011). When presented with this form, some parents may refuse to sign it. This refusal can also be documented.

A parent's decision not to vaccinate their child may not only impact their child, but also the community. If another person is harmed by a parent's failure to vaccinate, it has been suggested that the parent could be held liable in these situations (Diekema 2009).

References

American Academy of Pediatrics and the United States Public Health Service (1999) Joint statement of the American Academy of Pediatrics (AAP) and the United States Public Health Service (USPHS). Pediatrics 104(3):568–569

American Congress of Obstetricians and Gynecologists (ACOG) (2014) Reducing your risk of birth defects. http://www.acog.org/~/media/For%20Patients/faq146.pdf?dmc=1&ts=2014032 8T1436440030. Accessed 28 March 2014

American Medical Association. Report of the council on ethical and judicial affairs: pediatric decision-making. Published 2007. www.ama-assn.org/ama1/pub/upload/mm/369/ceja_8i07. pdf. Accessed March 10, 2014

Andrews N, Miller E, Grant A et al (2004) Thimerosal exposure in infants and developmental disorders: a retrospective cohort study in the United Kingdom does not support a causal association. Pediatrics 11:584–591

Atwell J, Van Otterloo J, Zipprich J et al (2013) Nonmedical vaccine exemptions and pertussis in California, 2010. Pediatrics 132:624–630

Birnbaum M, Jacobs E, Ralston-King J et al (2013) Correlates of high vaccination exemption rates among kindergartens. Vaccine 31:750–756

Blank N, Caplain A, Constable C (2013) Exempting schoolchildren from immunizations: states with few barriers had highest rates of nonmedical exemptions. Health Aff 32(7):1282–1290

Boylston A, Williams A (2008) Zabdiel Boylston's evaluation of inoculation against smallpox. J R Soc Med 101:527

Boylston Z (1726) An historical account of the smallpox inoculated in New England upon all sorts of persons, whites, blacks, and of all ages and constitution. S. Chandler, London

Bratton G (2011) Autism: what's the truth? http://blogs.jwatch.org/general-medicine/index. php/2011/01/autism-whats-the-truth/

Centers for Disease Control and Prevention (1999) Ten great public health achievements, 1900–1999: impact of vaccines universally recommended for children. Morb Mortal Wkly Rep 48(12):241–243

Centers for Disease Control and Prevention (2008) Outbreak of measles—San Diego, California, January–February 2008. Morb Mortal Wkly Rep 57(08):203–206

Centers for Disease Control and Prevention (2011) Measles—United States, January–May 20, 2011. Morb Mortal Wkly Rep 60(20):666–668

Centers for Disease Control and Prevention (2012) Epidemiology and prevention of vaccine-preventable diseases, 12th edn, second printing. Public Health Foundation, Washington DC (Atkinson W, Wolfe S, Hamborsky J, eds.)

Centers for Disease Control and Prevention (2013) Measles—United States, January 1–August 24, 2013. Morb Mortal Wkly Rep 62(36):741–743

Centers for Disease Control and Prevention (2013) Vaccination coverage among children in kindergarten—United States, 2012–2013 school year. Morb Mortal Wkly Rep 62(30):607–612

J. A. Boom, R. M. Cunningham, *Understanding and Managing Vaccine Concerns,* SpringerBriefs in Public Health, DOI 10.1007/978-3-319-07563-1, © Springer International Publishing Switzerland 2014

Cunningham R, Boom J (2013) Telling stories of vaccine-preventable diseases: why it works. S D Med spec no: 21–26

Dales L, Hammer S, Smith N (2001) Time trends in autism and in MMR immunization coverage in California. JAMA 285:1183–1185

Deer B (2011) Secrets of the MMR scare. BMJ 342:5347

Diekema D (2004) Parental refusals of medical treatment: the harm principle as threshold for state intervention. Theor Med Bioeth 25(4):243–264

Diekema D (2005) Responding to parental refusals of immunization of children. Pediatrics 115(5):1428–1431

Diekema D (2009) Choices should have consequences: failure to vaccinate, harm to others, and civil liability. Mich Rev Law First Impressions 107:90

Diekema D, Kamin D, Kesselheim J (2012) Parents refuse vaccines? Ethical response needed. Med Ethics Adv 28(9):106–107

Diekema D (2013) Provider dismissal of vaccine-hesitant families: misguided policy that fails to benefit children. Hum Vaccin Immunother 9(12):1–2

Ernst K, Jacobs E (2012) Implications of philosophical and personal belief exemptions on re-emergence of vaccine-preventable disease: the role of spatial clustering in under-vaccination. Hum Vaccin Immunother 8(6):838–841

Farrington CP, Miller E, Taylor B (2001) MMR and autism: further evidence against a causal association. Vaccine 19:3632–3635

Feikin D, Lezotte D, Hamman R et al (2000) Individual and community risks of measles and pertussis associated with personal exemptions to immunization. JAMA 282(24):3145–3150

Fernbach A (2011) Parental rights and decision making regarding vaccinations: ethical dilemmas for the primary care provider. J Am Acad Nurse Pract 23:336–345

Fine P (2004) Vaccines, 4th edn. Philadelphia

Flanagan-Klygis E, Sharp L, Frader J (2005) Dismissing the family who refuses vaccines. Arch Pediatr Adoles Med 159:929–934

Fombonne E, Zakarian R, Bennett A et al (2006) Pervasive developmental disorders in Montreal, Quebec, Canada: prevalence and links with immunizations. Pediatrics 118:e139–e150

Frederickson D, Davis T, Arnold C et al (2004) Childhood immunization refusal: provider and parent perceptions. Fam Med 36(6):431–439

Freed G, Clark S, Butchart A, Singer D, Davis M (2010) Parental vaccine safety concerns in 2009. Pediatrics 125:654–659

Gaudino J, Robison S (2012) Risk factors associated with parents claiming personal-belief exemptions to school immunization requirements: community and other influences on more skeptical parents in Oregon, 2006. Vaccine 30:1132–1142

Gellin B, Maibach E, Marcuse E (2000) Do parents understand immunizations? A national telephone survey. Pediatrics 106(5):1097–1102

Gilmour J, Harrison C, Asadi L et al (2011) Childhood immunizations: when physicians and parents disagree. Pediatrics 128:S167–S174

Glanz J, McClure D, Magid D et al (2009) Parental refusal of pertussis vaccination is associated with an increased risk of pertussis infection in children. Pediatrics 123:1446–1451

Glanz J, McClure D, Magid D (2010) Parental refusal of varicella vaccination and the associated risk of varicella infection in children. Arch Pediatr Adolesc Med 164(1):66–69

Glanz J, McClure D, O'Leary S et al (2011) Parental decline of pneumococcal vaccination and risk of pneumococcal related disease in children. Vaccine 29:994–999

Glass R, Parashar U (2014) Rotavirus vaccines—balancing intussusception risks and health benefits. N Engl J Med 370(6):568–570

Goldstein J (1977) Medical care for the child at risk: on state supervention of parental autonomy. Yale Law J 86(4):645–670

Gust D, Brown C, Sheedy K et al (2005) Immunization attitudes and beliefs among parents: beyond a dichotomous perspective. Am J Health Behav 29(1):81–92

Gust D, Darling N, Kennedy A et al (2008) Parents with doubts about vaccines: which vaccines and reasons why. Pediatrics 122:718–725

Gust D, Woodruff R, Kennedy A (2003) Parental perceptions surrounding risks and benefits of immunization. Semin Pediatr Infect Dis 14(3):207–212

Hammond B, Sipics M, Youngdahl K (2013) The history of vaccines. Philadelphia

Heron J, Golding J (2004) Thimerosal exposure in infants and developmental disorders: a prospective cohort study in the United Kingdom does not support a causal association. Pediatrics 114:577–583

Hviid A, Stellfeld M, Wohlfahrt J et al (2003) Association between thimerosal-containing vaccine and autism. JAMA 290:1763–1766

Immunization AC (2013) Personal belief exemptions for vaccination put people at risk. Examine the evidence for yourself. http://www.immunize.org/catg.d/p2069.pdf. Accessed 14 March 2014

Jacobsen R, Van Etta L, Bahta L (2013) The C.A.S.E. approach: guidance for talking to vaccine-hesitant parents. Minn Medicine: 49–50

Kamin D (2012) Is vaccine refusal reason to terminate relationship? Med Ethics Adv 28(12):143

Kaye J, del Mar Melero-Montes M, Jick H (2001) Mumps, measles, and rubella vaccine and the incidence of autism recorded by general practitioners: a time trend analysis. BMJ 322:460–463

Kempe A, Daley M, McCauley M et al (2011) Prevalence of parental concerns about childhood vaccines: the experience of primary care physicians. Am J Prev Med 40(5):548–555

Leask J, Kinnersley P, Jackson C et al (2012) Communicating with parents about vaccination: a framework for health professionals. BMC Pediatr 12:154

Lieb S, Liberators P, Edwards K (2011) Pediatricians' experience with and response to parental vaccine safety concerns and vaccine refusal: a survey of Connecticut pediatricians. Public Health Rep 126(2):13–23

Madsen K, Hviid A, Vestergaard M et al (2002) A population-based study of measles, mumps, and rubella vaccination and autism. N Engl J Med 347:1477–1482

Madsen K, Lauritsen M, Pedersen C et al (2003) Thimerosal and the occurrence of autism: negative ecological evidence from Danish population-based data. Pediatrics 112:604–606

Mayhew A, Mullins T, Ding L (2014) Risk perceptions and subsequent sexual behaviors after HPV vaccination in adolescents. Pediatrics 133:404–411

National Humanities Center (2009) National Humanities Center Resource Toolbox. http://nationalhumanitiescenter.org/pds/becomingamer/ideas/text7/smallpoxvaccination.pdf/. Accessed 13 March 2014

National Research Council (2004) Immunization safety review: vaccines and autism. The National Academies, Washington, D.C

Offit P, Moser C (2009) The problem with Dr. Bob's alternative vaccine schedule. Pediatrics 123:e164–e169

Offit P, Moser C (2011) Vaccines and your child: separating fact from fiction. New York

Offit P (2011) Deadly choices: how the anti-vaccine movement threatens us all. New York

Offit P (2005) The Cutter incident: how America's first polio vaccine led to the growing vaccine crisis.Connecticut, New Haven

Omer S, Enger K, Moulton L et al (2008) Geographic clustering of nonmedical exemptions to school immunization requirements and associations with geographic clustering of pertussis. Am J Epidemiol 168:1389–1396

Omer S, Pan W, Halsey N et al (2006) Nonmedical exemptions to school immunization requirements: secular trends and association of state policies with pertussis incidence. JAMA 296(14):1757–1763

Omer S, Richards J, Ward M et al (2012) Vaccination policies and rates of exemption from immunization, 2005-2011. N Engl J Med 367(12):1170–1171

Omer S, Salmon D, Orenstein W et al (2009) Vaccine refusal, mandatory immunization, and the risks of vaccine-preventable diseases. N Engl J Med 360(19):1981–1988

Opel D, Feemster K, Omer S et al (2014) A 6-month old with vaccine-hesitant parents. Pediatrics 133:526–530

Opel D, Heritage J, Taylor J et al (2013) The architecture of provider-parent vaccine discussions at health supervision visits. Pediatrics 132(6):1–10

Orenstein W, Hinman A (1999) The immunization system in the United States—the role of school immunization law. Vaccine 17:S19–S24

Peltola H, Patja A, Leinikki P et al (1998) No evidence for measles, mumps, and rubella vaccine associated inflammatory bowel disease or autism in a 14-year prospective study. The Lancet 351:1327–1328

Richards J, Wagenaar B, Otterloo J et al (2013) Nonmedical exemptions to immunization requirements in California: a 16-year longitudinal analysis of trends and associated community factors. Vaccine 31:3009–3013

Ropeik D (2006) How Americans are living dangerously. Time magazine

Salmon D, Haber M, Gangarosa E et al (1999) Health consequences of religious and philosophical exemptions from immunization laws. JAMA 281(1):47–53

Salmon D, Moulton L, Omer S et al (2005) Factors associated with refusal of childhood vaccines among parents of school-aged children: a case-control study. Arch Pediatr Adolesc Med 159:470–476

Schwartz J, Caplan A (2011) Vaccination refusal: ethics, individual rights, and the common good. Prim Care Clin Office Pract 38:717–728

Sears R (2011) The vaccine book: making the right decision for your child. New York

Shui I, Weintraub E, Gus D (2006) Parents concerned about vaccine safety: differences in race/ethnicity and attitudes. Am J Prev Med 31(3):244–251

Smith P, Chu S, Barker L (2004) Children who have received no vaccines: who are they and where do they live? Pediatrics 114:187–195

Smith P, Humiston S, Marcuse E et al (2011) Parental delay or refusal of vaccine doses, childhood vaccination coverage at 24 months of age, and the health belief model. Public Health Rep 126(2):135–146

Stehr-Green P, Tull P, Stellfeld M et al (2003) Autism and thimerosal-containing vaccines: lack of consistent evidence for an association. Am J Prev Med 25:101–106

Taylor B, Miller E, Farrington CP et al (1999) Autism and measles, mumps, and rubella vaccine: no epidemiological evidence for a causal association. The Lancet 353:2026–2029

Taylor B, Miller E, Lingam R et al (2002) Measles, mumps, and rubella vaccination and bowel problems or developmental regression in children with autism: population study. BMJ 324:393–396

Verstraeten T, Davis R, DeStefano F et al (2003) Safety of thimerosal-containing vaccines: a two-phased study of computerized health maintenance organization databases. Pediatrics 112:1039–1048

Wakefield A, Murch S, Anthony A et al (1998) Retracted: Illeal-lymphoid-nodular hyperplasia, non-specific colitis, and pervasive developmental disorder in children. The Lancet 351:637–641

Index

J. A. Boom, R. M. Cunningham, *Understanding and Managing Vaccine Concerns,*   41
SpringerBriefs in Public Health, DOI 10.1007/978-3-319-07563-1,
© Springer International Publishing Switzerland 2014

CPSIA information can be obtained at www.ICGtesting.com
Printed in the USA
LVOW12s1829310714

396939LV00007B/404/P